Knowing More about the Ear

Treating Deafness and other Maladies of the Ear

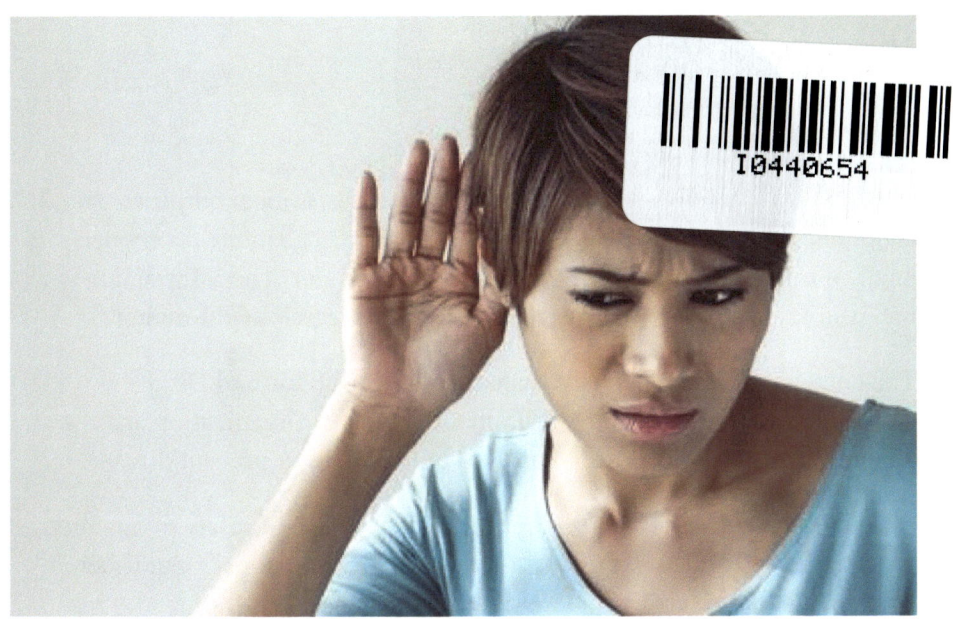

Dueep Jyot Singh

Science of Living Series

Mendon Cottage Books

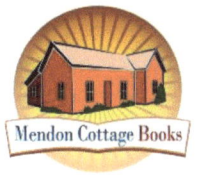

JD-Biz Publishing

Download Free Books!

http://MendonCottageBooks.com

All Rights Reserved.

No part of this publication may be reproduced in any form or by any means, including scanning, photocopying, or otherwise without prior written permission from JD-Biz Corp Copyright © 2015

All Images Licensed by Fotolia and 123RF.

Disclaimer

The information is this book is provided for informational purposes only. It is not intended to be used and medical advice or a substitute for proper medical treatment by a qualified health care provider. The information is believed to be accurate as presented based on research by the author.

The contents have not been evaluated by the U.S. Food and Drug Administration or any other Government or Health Organization and the contents in this book are not to be used to treat cure or prevent disease.

The author or publisher is not responsible for the use or safety of any diet, procedure or treatment mentioned in this book. The author or publisher is not responsible for errors or omissions that may exist.

Warning

The Book is for informational purposes only and before taking on any diet, treatment or medical procedure, it is recommended to consult with your primary health care provider.

Our books are available at

1. Amazon.com
2. Barnes and Noble
3. Itunes
4. Kobo
5. Smashwords
6. Google Play Books

Download Free Books!

http://MendonCottageBooks.com

Table of Contents

Introduction

One of the basic tenets of good health is that you have all your five senses in perfect working condition. These include vision, smell, hearing, touch and taste. That is the reason why responsible parents need to make sure that their children do not suffer from any sort of ear maladies which can possibly lead to deafness as time goes by.

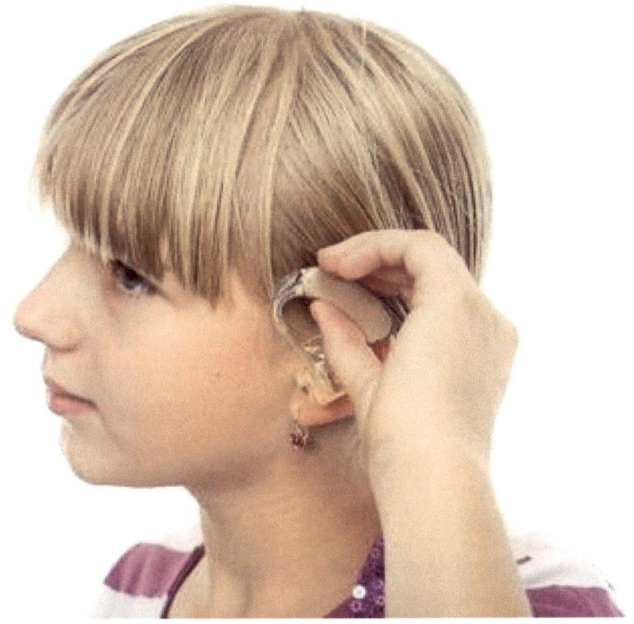

I remember taking over a teaching job temporarily for a friend, more than two decades ago. I had to take care of three year old nursery children which was about as perilous a job, as one could ever wish for. Now there was this very bright-eyed little baby boy, who had never spoken a word. His parents were identified that he was deaf, but they had got his ears checked up, to make sure that he was not suffering from any possible birth defects.

Three years old, not one peep and not one sound out of him, it was worrying. Until one fine afternoon, he announced to his parents that they had better ask me to be his teacher and his teacher alone because he did not want to share me with the rest of his classmates!

When his nearly tearful father asked him why he had not spoken for all these years, he said very practically, that they had made sure that he did not need to talk ever because all his needs were fulfilled. Besides that, they did all the talking all the time so why did he need to talk?

This young gentleman is now at college, and one cannot stop him talking. He has a keen debater and intends to argue the point on every small matter whenever he can, However, he can whenever he can. When once I recounted to him episodes in the life and times off a three-year-old, he gives me a "Come off It Ma'am" look. He never talk? Not going to happen.

When I was a little child my grandfather often told me about a ritual which the elders practice whenever a child was born. They rang the silver bell behind him, to bring all the good spirits near the new born child to bless it. And if the child followed the sound of the bell, they would consider that it would live a good and virtuous life. According to me, this was the way in which they managed to find out whether the child was not suffering from congenital deafness. Also, I keep wondering about those poor little children, who were scared out of their diapers with that harsh clanging noise however much their elders considered it to be musical.

The bell was rung over me, when I was born. According to my grandfather I heard it and set up a howl fit to burst the eardrums of everybody in the vicinity and got all the nurses running to soothe me. This not only proved that I was able to hear, but I was also going to be a potential critic of all the idiotic actions adults did in the future.

So this book is going to tell you all about your ears, how to take care of them, and some ailments of the ears, which can be treated either naturally, or by your doctors.

The Construction of the Ear

The ear consists of three regions- the external ear, the middle ear and the inner ear. The external ear consists of the Pinna and the ear canal. The ear canal is responsible for transmitting sound waves to the eardrum of the middle ear.

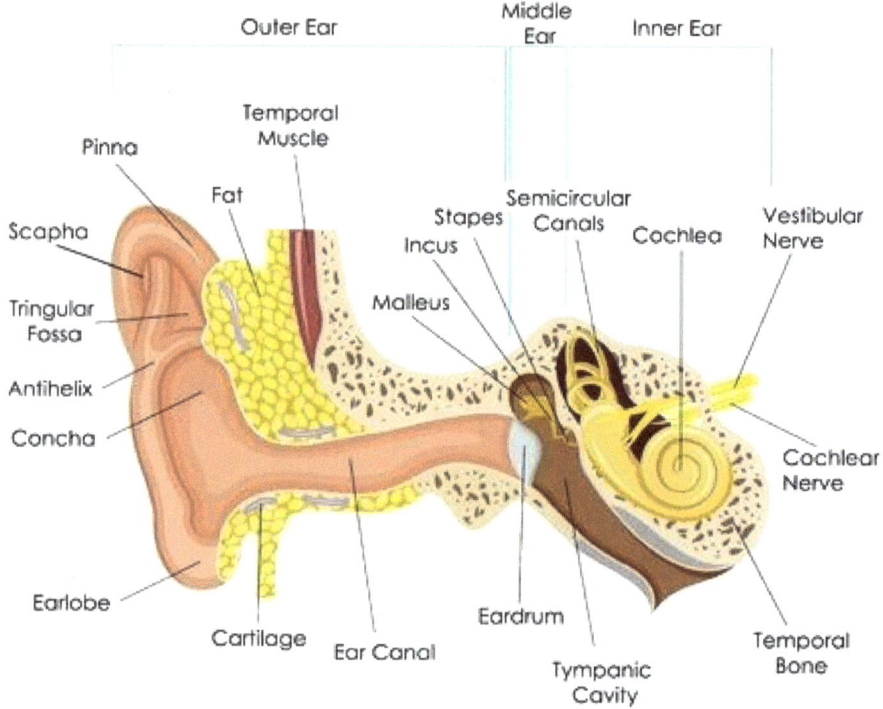

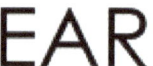

EAR

There are 3 small bones in the middle ear. They are called ossicles. These vibrate with the sound waves which are then transmitted further onwards to the inner ear.

The middle ear is connected to the nose through the eustachian tube which equalizes the pressure on both sides of the eardrum.

The inner ear consists of the shell -shaped cochlea.

The ear also has a vestibule which has three semicircular canals. These maintain the balance of the body. The inner ear is connected to the brain by the auditory nerve. It analyzes the sound. It is what tells the brain that these noises that are being heard are terribly loud, discordant, and are going to cause a splitting headache, if there is too much of continual exposure to that same noisy environment. The final hearing occurs in the brain, through the auditory nerves.

Symptoms of Hearing Problems

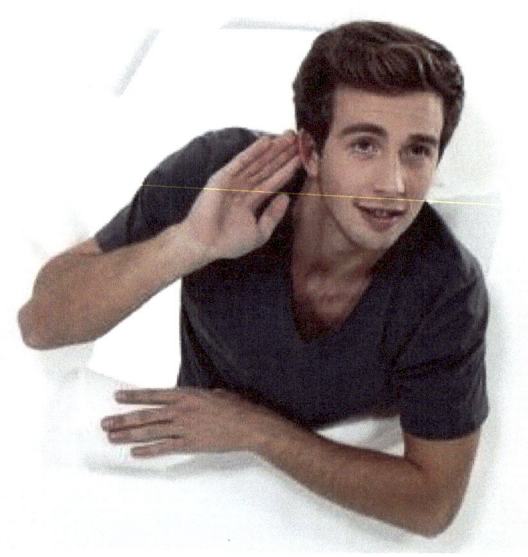

The clichéd hand behind the ear pinna and an open mouth saying "What?" in a querying tone may look amusing once in a while, but when it is repeated too often, it means that the hearer is suffering from hearing problems. Recognition of this particular problem is the first step in rectifying it.

Some of the common signs indicating hearing problems are going to include

Inability to hear high-pitched voices like those of children and some women. With the passing of age, my father suffers from hearing problems, and as he is surrounded by his grandchildren and women, – I included, he keeps telling us to speak in lower pitches. That means we have to deepen our voices when we talk to him.

He could use a hearing aid in order to hear more clearly, but he does not want to be dependent on such artificial and scientific complex gadgets. But then hearing aids are necessary, especially when a person grows older. But as my father is fond of recounting an old chestnut, someone asked an old millionaire how he liked his new hearing aid, which he had bought, without the knowledge of his family members. Wonderful, he said, I have already changed my Will thrice.

Also, if you find difficulty in hearing at public gatherings, theater, etc. where the source of the sound is distant, you may need to get your ears checked.

In the same manner, if you find difficulty in understanding conversations and following them within the group of people all speaking at different pitches and tones, that is a sign that your hearing is deteriorating. In the same way, if you find it difficult to follow what is being said on the TV [this is mostly going to be the actors saying "We Have To Talk", if you are listening to the long winded family serials where people are murdered regularly and turn up hale and hearty after 10 episodes on frantic public demand.]

Common Problems of the Ear

Some of the more common ailments which affect your ear are –

Deafness, infections in the ear – causing discharge, pain in the ear, giddiness or vertigo and Tintinnus.

Deafness

Deafness is normally caused by diseases and infections in one or more parts of the ear.

The problems faced by infections in your external ear include wax, fungus, foreign bodies, and acute infection.

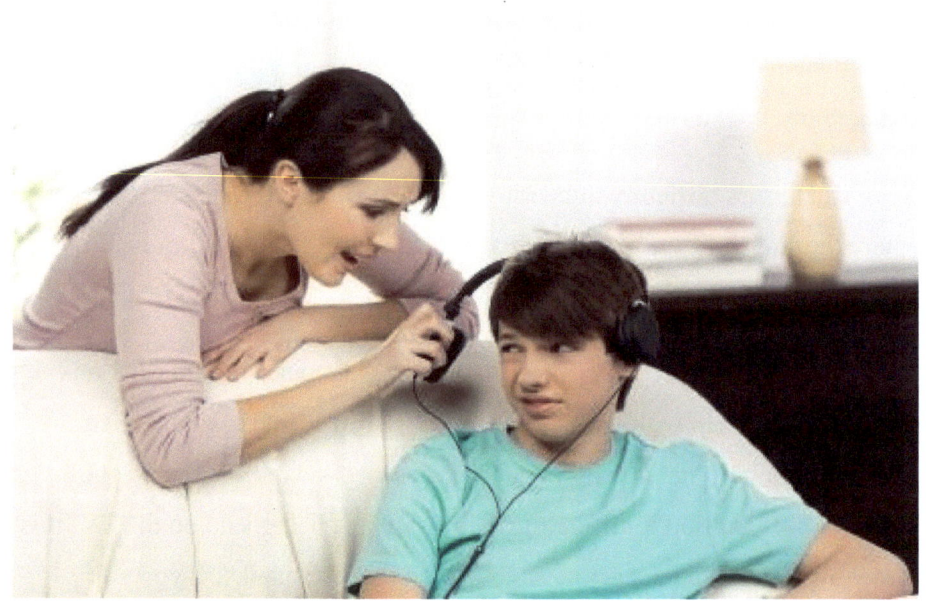

Too much loud music can also cause deafness.

When I was a child, I suffered terribly from otitis externa. This meant that every third day, there would be a painful deposit in my ear, which had to be cleared out at the base hospital. The doctor who happened to be a bit of a supposed wit and wag, used to call it a Swiss bank deposit, with all that accumulation gathering there and multiplying.

The reason was because there were two factors promoting this ear infection. We lived in an area which was humid and moist. Also, I couldn't resist spending a major part of the day in the swimming pool, in our house. The water was definitely not hygienic, clear or sanitary there, because most of the time it was filled up with rainwater.

So in I used to go in that water, do my bit of swimming, and come out with my ears wet. No wonder the fungus or the bacterial infections flourished there. Nobody told me to dry the inside of my ears, after I had come out from the water.

And so every third day, I would be yelling with pain, because my ears ached so terribly and had to get them cleaned out by Dr. M. And then he would give me some eardrops to put in my ears, three times a day, in order to get rid of the fungal infection.

But he didn't know that this infection had no chance of clearing up, because the moment I came back from the hospital, I would go right into the swimming pool, showing off splaaaashing around.

It was only when my grandmother got really tired of my waking up at night, holding my ears and yowling like a scalded cat, that she tried out one of her natural remedy recipes. She burned some cloves of crushed garlic in some mustard oil[1] and put the still warm drops in my ears. She cleaned out the infection after three hours. And then she put the drops in again.

---

[1] Traditionally this remedy is made with mustard oil, garlic and a touch of "sindoor". https://en.wikipedia.org/wiki/Sindoor This is a mixture is traditionally made up of Alum or lime, and I wouldn't be surprised that the alum helped in the curing of the fungal infections.

Nowadays, this item available in the market is heavily adulterated with red lead, so if you want to try out this remedy to get rid of your infections, never use sindoor in it, unless you have a friend making it for you traditionally!

Two days of this cure, and the infection which had tormented me for the past 2 ½ years cleared out, never to come back, even though I never gave up my swimming to this day.

So if you have any sort of discharge coming out from your years, this can because due to fungus and acute infection of the external ear.

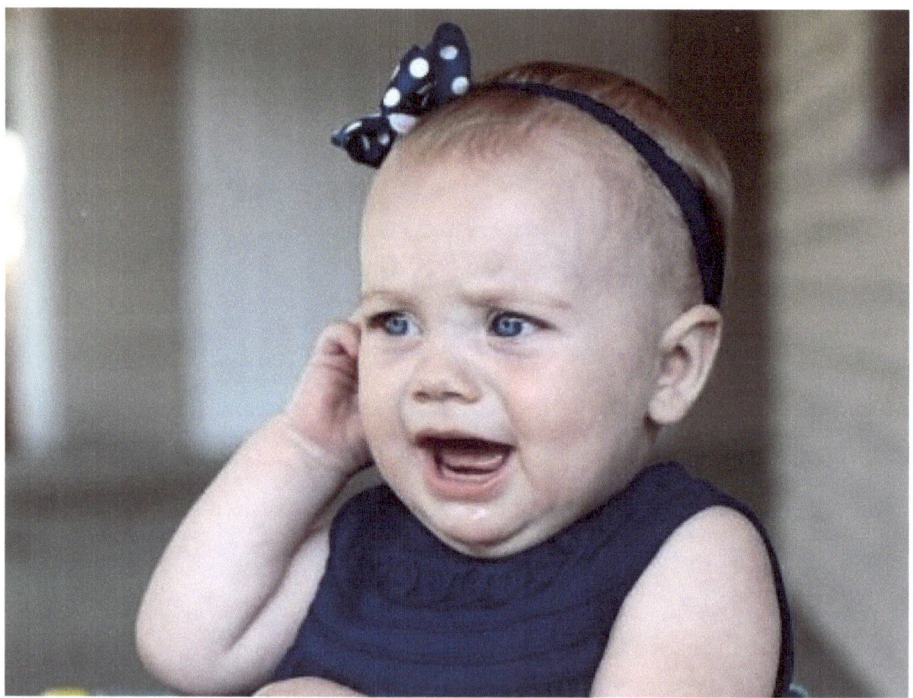

Middle Ear Problems

Persistant or occasional infections in your middle ear, or collection of fluid in the ears, known as otosclerosis, causing spongy bone growth, can lead to deafness in the ear.

Cholestetoma

Perforation, or a whole, in the ear drum can also cause deafness. If these perforations are located in the upper or smaller areas of the ear drum, this can lead to a dangerous condition known as cholestetoma. The bone surrounding this area is going to erode slowly, which will lead to other issues. Dizziness, infection in the mastoid area (bony protuberance found behind the ear), facial paralysis, possible abscess in the brain, and meningitis, are all possible side effects.

Perforations, for the most part, are usually benign, and are not likely to result in these dangerous complications. They will, however, cause deafness and occasional discharge from the ear.

Ear Perforations

Perforations lasting only a short time may just heal themselves, which is the case the majority of the time. One will need to go to an Ear Nose Throat (ENT) specialist, if the perforation has not healed in 6 to 8 weeks. Usually one of two options occur, first, for small perforations, the doctor will close it by using chemical cautery. For larger perforations, or a failed chemical cautery, the doctor may perform a tympanoplasty. This is where they use a surgical microscope to place a paper patch. Both of these methods are used for benign perforations only.

Ear discharge is normally treated medically and surgically in the first instance, infection can be controlled by antibiotics which are given orally, and an antibiotic or antiseptic ear drops, along with the care of the ear, followed strictly. This was what Dr. M did for me, cleaning out my ear every three days, after he thought the fungal infection was being controlled with ear drops.

In the same way fungal infections are treated with antifungal eardrops and oral antibiotics.

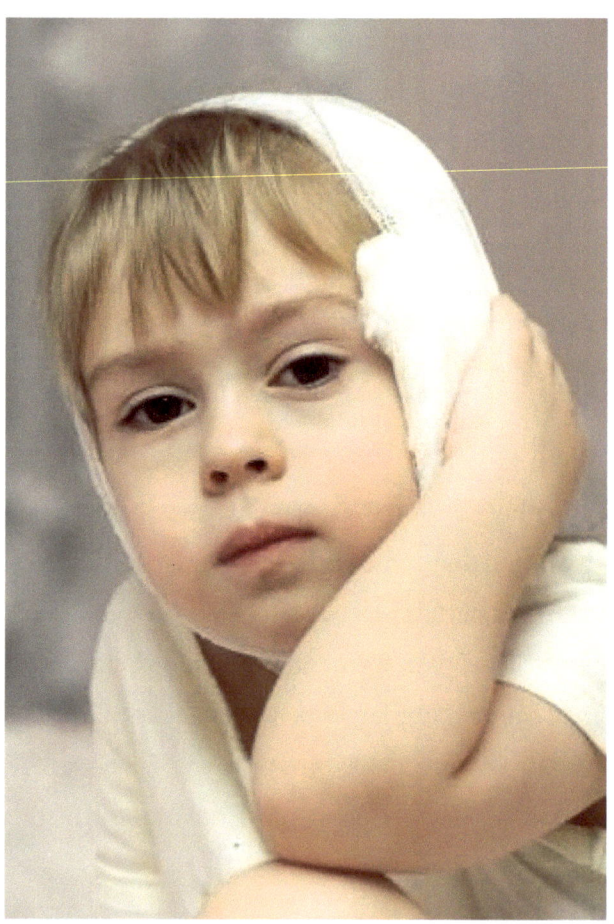

Inner Ear Problems

There are many causes of ear problems: birth defects, infections, uncontrolled blood pressure, diabetes, injuries, tumor in the auditory nerve, diseases causing vertigo (i.e. Meniere's disease), aging, and noise inducing deafness.

I remember as a child, feeling amused at one of our playmates, who could not walk a straight line. The youngster put his hands out, and always lost his balance. It was later we found out that he had ear problems, which prevented him from keeping his balance. He also suffered from vertigo and that is why we were rather cruel and played on the really high rooftops, whenever we didn't want him around.

Pain in the Ear

This is such a common malady that in ancient times, whenever anybody suffered from any sort of earache, the woman of the house just heated up an onion, wrapped it up in a piece of flannel, and tied the onion to the affected ear. This heat therapy cause the pain to go away, in many cases unless, of course, the ear was infected very badly. That was when the barber or the nearest apothecary was called to try his own quackery to get rid of the ear ache.

There are a number of reasons and causes of pain apart from infection in the middle and external ear.

"Referred pain"

There is one surprising cause of pain, known as referred pain. The ear has an immense nerve supply. Your tongue, teeth, cheek, jaw joint, throat, and the neck are all supplied from these nerves.

Any sort of pain in this area maybe interpreted as pain in the ear, because the ear is such a sensitive structure. For example, if one is suffering from jaw pain, one may also feel like they are suffering from an earache too!

Neuralgic Pain

This normally occurs due to oversensitive nerves. It was quite a fashionable malady, especially with ladies in Regency times, when they pretended that it was stylish to suffer from neuralgic pain. Their sensibilities were so delicate and tender. Their nerves were supposedly very sensitive and prone to breakdowns. That is why, they suffered from what they could termed as "neuralgia". All this was an affectation and psychosomatic. Real neurologic pain is painful, because after all, it is in your nerves.

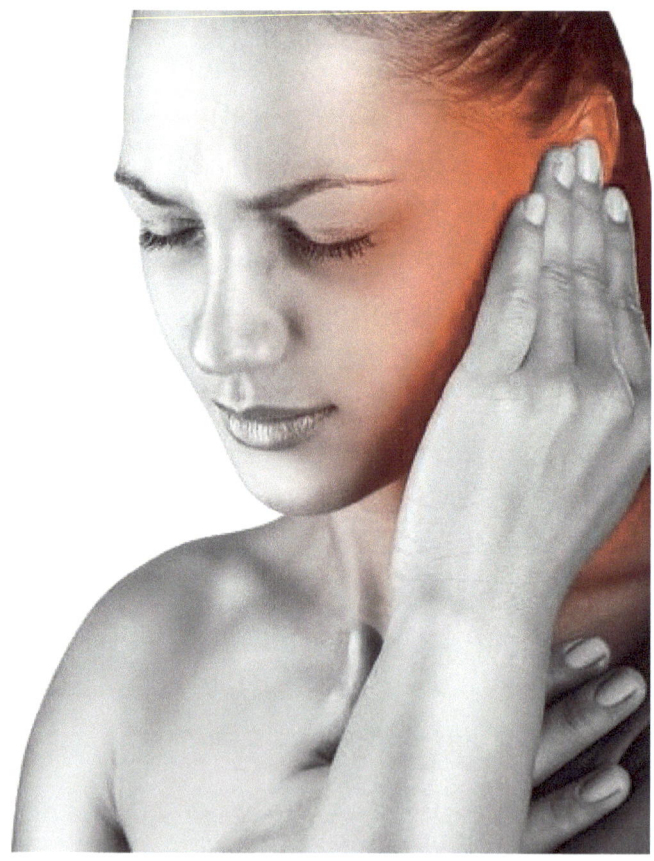

You can get symptomatic relief from earache through painkillers. You can also ferment the ear with a hot water bottle or a fomenting pad. The onion of yore did the same job of fomentation down the ages.

It is necessary that you get your ears checked up by an ENT surgeon immediately, the moment you feel pain in your ear under any circumstances or situations. You do not want them infected, do you.

Giddiness/vertigo

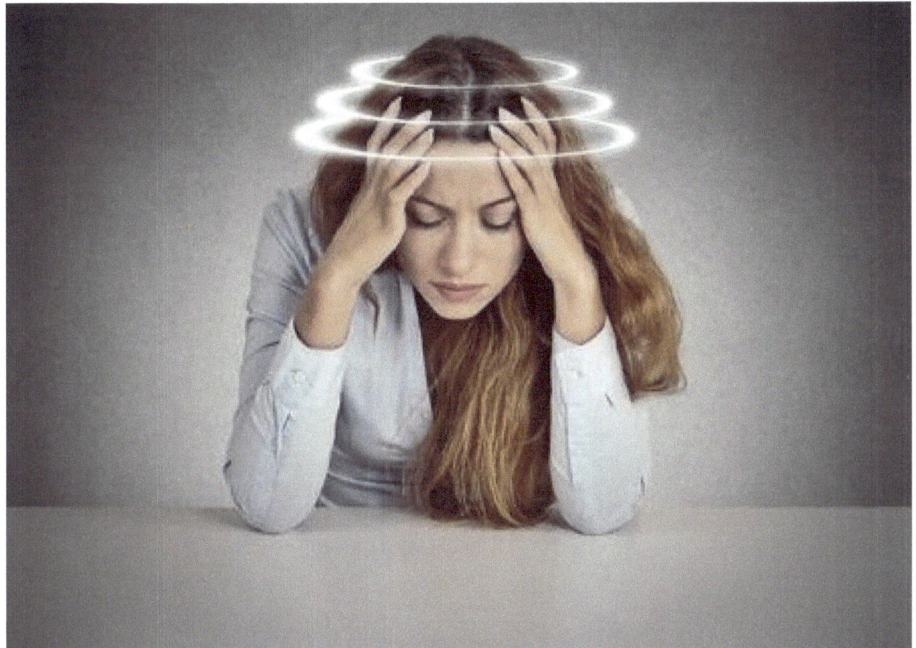

Many people confuse giddiness and nausea, there is a difference. Nausea is normally caused from side effects of a medication, ill health, and possibly food poisoning. Giddiness, on the other hand, is when you feel dizzy, or when one cannot walk properly, this usually involves staggering and falling. One can also have a whirling sensation inside one's head. Giddiness can also be caused due to exposure in the sun. This is going to be accompanied by nausea, when you find yourself up- chucking your breakfast. Incidentally, in cases of migraine, clearing out your system gets rid of the giddiness too.

If you are feeling giddy or suffer from vertigo, there is a chance that you may be suffering from some ear ailments. That is because two functions happen in the inner ear. This includes the hearing of sounds, by the cochlear part (a spiral structure, looking like a snail shell, in the inner ear) and by the vestibular part (the middle cavity of the inner ear between the cochlea and the semicircular canals), which keeps the maintenance of the balance. Lesions (wounds) which are affecting the vestibular part may also cause giddiness.

Also, if you are suffering from diseases like high or low BP, diabetes, tumors, anemia and other related problems, these can also cause vertigo. Mental stress can also aggravate any case of vertigo. Your ENT surgeon is best equipped to diagnose the cause and treatment of giddiness.

Tinnitus

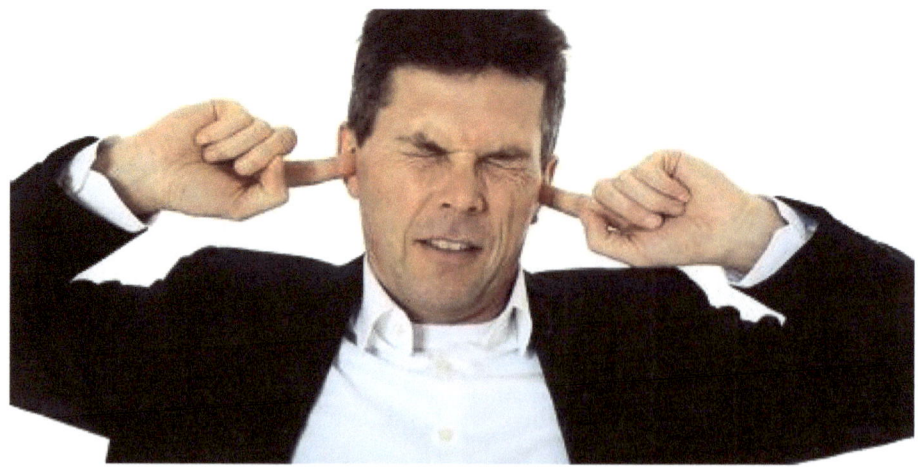

If you are suffering from noises in the ear or in the head, this tends to become very annoying. This is known as tinnitus and is normally caused by diseases in the ear or outside the ear. So what are the noises going to sound like, if you have never experienced it before?

Just imagine picking up a seashell and placing it in front of your ears. You are going to hear a sound, as if the seashell is remembering the sounds of the waves. Actually, the sounds are all manufactured in the ear itself, and this noise in the head or in the ear, magnified greatly is called tinnitus.

You may also feel that there is the sound of drumbeats pounding in your head.

Tinnitus may persist even after you have got the disease, which caused the tinnitus cured properly. This can be disturbing. In such cases, the patient may need a psychiatric opinion and help. They may recommend tinnitus maskers to you.

These maskers are similar to hearing aids, and generate continuous noise based on the fact that the patient is more comfortable in a noisy environment than in quiet surroundings.

Getting Your Hearing Tested

If you suspect any sort of hearing loss, you need to get an examination done by a doctor who specializes in ENT. He is going to test your hearing and evaluate its possible deterioration. A short and simple test, which is called an audiometry, is going to determine the type and the severity of hearing loss.

My father got this audiometry test done a couple of years ago, when he was around 82 years of age. He came back home, really happy because the doctor had said that he suffered only from 70% hearing loss! That means that he could hear 30% and he did not need any hearing aid yet!

After the age of 50, a hearing test has to be taken regularly. Along with the physical checkup, one would want to get your doctor to do an audiometry test, especially if one is suffering from ringing in the ears.

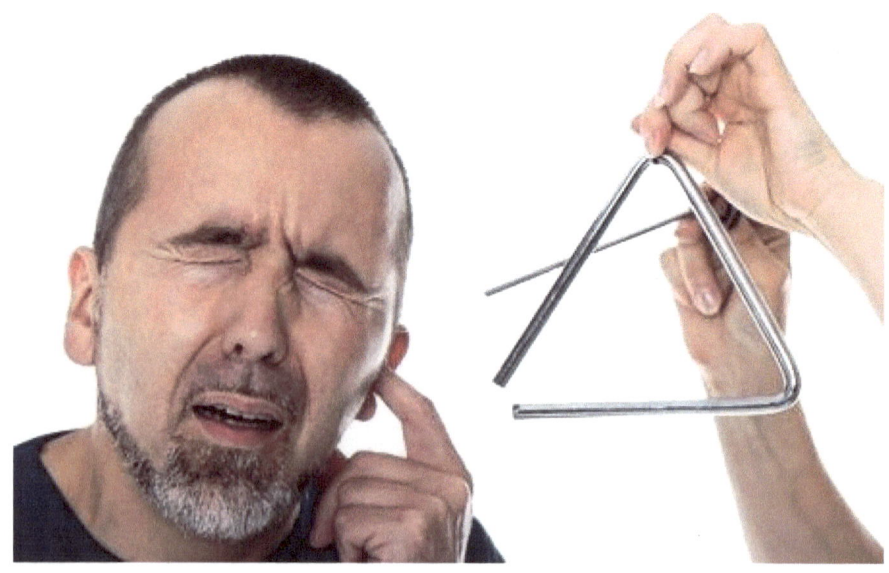

Types of Hearing Loss

After your hearing has been tested by the ENT specialist, he is going to determine the type and degree of the hearing loss. This is done by studying the graphic record made, as part of the hearing test.

An injury or problem, in the bones, membranes, or eardrum can cause

conductive hearing loss.

This particular hearing loss can usually be overcome by medication or surgery.

Sensorineural Hearing Loss

If one has sensorineural hearing loss, which is deafness of the inner ear, it is going to be rather difficult to treat. That is because it is caused by the deterioration of the inner ear or the auditory nerves.

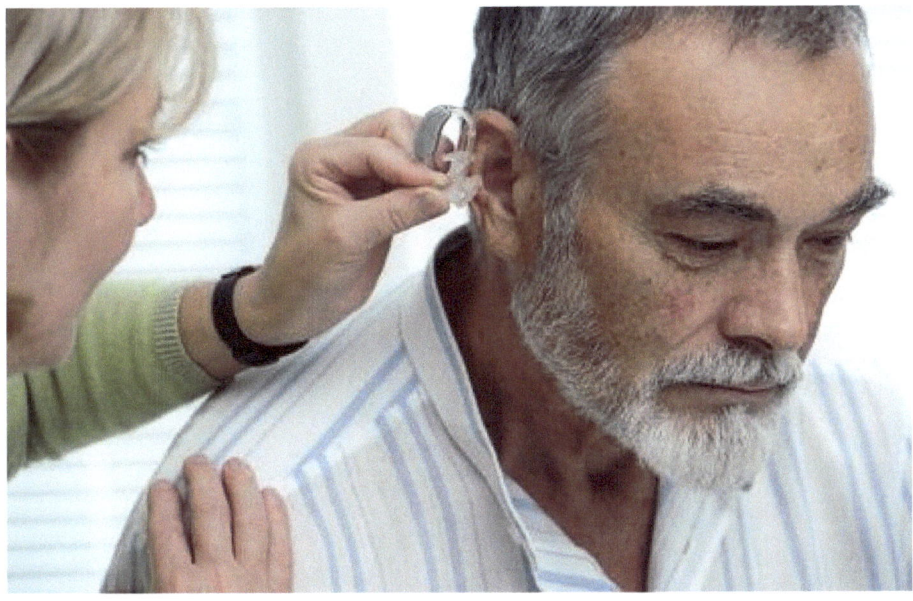

If this is the case, the doctors are going to prescribe hearing aids for you because that is the only reasonable solution available. In profound deafness, a cochlear implant may also be considered.

You may also suffered from mixed hearing loss, which is a combination of both conductive hearing and sensorineural hearing.

Can Deafness Be Cured?

With the advance of scientific treatment methods, and technology, the diseases of the external and middle ear – conductive deafness – can be treated with medical treatments and surgery. Also, diseases like were rations in the eardrum or fixation of the innermost small bone in the middle ear can be treated surgically.

These procedures are called tympanoplasty and stapedectomy with the use of Teflon piston grafting.

Let me talk a bit about the eardrum also known as the tympanum. When I was suffering from Otitis, as a child, Dr. M told me very strictly not to poke an earbud, however much I wished to, to get rid of the pain and irritation, because there was a possibility that I would burst my ear drum. And that would make me permanently deaf.

When I was at college, I fell down while training for intercollegiate games, and for a couple of days, I could not hear anything in my right ear. Oh man, I told myself, that is that, I am going to spend the rest of my life with one hand behind my right ear, and asking people to talk on my left side, so that I can hear them. I had a feeling that the eardrum had burst. Luckily that was not the case.

However, injuries can cause the tympanum to burst. I have heard of cases when the perforations in the tympanum healed themselves, but they are not so common. So naturally, you are going to take care of your ears, the way you take care of your eyes.

As all the structures of the ear are very small, surgery is normally done with the help of special binocular microscopes under good illumination and magnification. If it is done properly by an experienced surgeon, it is going to result in high degrees of success. These are some common surgical procedures which are being followed all over the world today, even though there are many other more sophisticated and expensive surgical procedures being followed by specialists in the UK, Japan and in the USA, today.

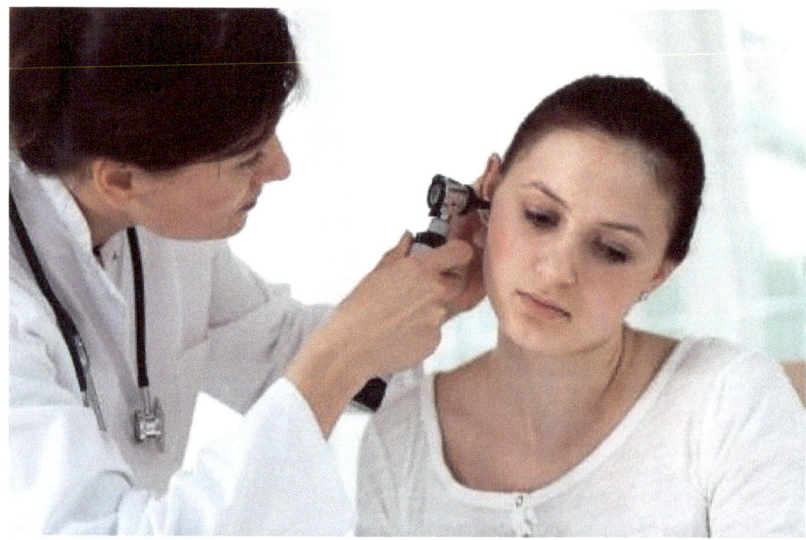

However, if you are suffering from sensorineural problems, like I said before, it is going to be very difficult to treat and you will have to resort to hearing aids.

How Does a Hearing Aid Work?

A hearing aid is an electronic device which magnifies sound selectively in various frequencies. After an audiogram is done by any ENT specialist, the patient is going to be recommended the best hearing aid which is going to matches his audiogram.

Remember to try it out for a few minutes before you buy it.

These hearing aids come in many shapes and sizes today. To have a better fitting, an ear mold in the shape of the ear of the patient is prepared for the hearing aid. Apart from the behind the ear hearing aids, you can get old fashioned pocket hearing aids, which you slip into your nearest pocket, and you have a hearing On button near to your hand, which you switch on whenever you want to listen to a conversation.

I remember my grand uncle being bought one of these pocket hearing aids about 30 years ago when behind the ear hearing aids were not so, nor en vogue. Even then, his family members found that it was very difficult to communicate with him. And soon they found that he did not switch on the hearing aid on purpose, because according to him, all he heard was people talking talking talking. He had been hearing that for the past 60 years, and he wanted some peace and quiet at his age. Now this is an amusing way in which one can console oneself for a hearing loss.

Even today, in his late 90s, he never switches on his hearing aid because the first thing that he is going to hear is how are you? And he is tired of hearing people ask him that!

Different models of hearing aids are going to remedy different types of hearing loss. Three types of hearing aids, – Completely in the Canal, CIC,

IN the Canal ITC and In the Ear ITE – are Custom-Designed to suit the requirements of the patients and their personal needs.

Behind the ear [BTE] hearing aids are attached to a customized ear mold. These can be modified so as to be compatible with external sound sources. That means you can hear training equipment, stereos, TV, radio, etc.. These are normally recommended for children and also those who require high amplification.

Pocket type hearing aid models are suited to young children and the elderly. That is because they have problems with dexterity, especially while trying to manipulate more sophisticated hearing aid models.

Computer Programmed and Digital Hearing Aids

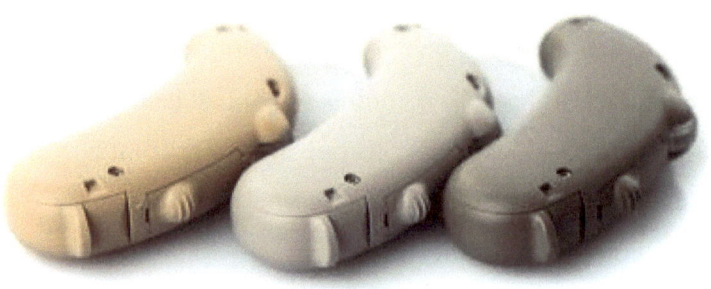

Digital and programmable computerized hearing aids are now coming into the market with more advanced technology and models available in CIC ITC ITE and BTE models, hearing aids are gaining a new life in efficiency.

Digital technology can enable you to hear loud and soft sounds. You can also hear high and low tones, practically at the level of a person with normal hearing.

Added to which, these hearing aids also have excellent speech intelligibility in noise. This means that   low-frequency noise like in a car or even in the aircraft is reduced and the clarity of speech is going to be enhanced to a pleasant level.

With these hearing aids, you are going to hear your environment just like you used to do, and you would like to, now. More and more individually adjustable hearing programs to provide this facility are coming in the market today.

For example, if you want a program which suits your working environment or home, you are not going to have any noise spoiling the hearing experience. Thanks to the latest technology, interference from cordless as well as mobile phones have also been cut drastically.

Cochlear Implants

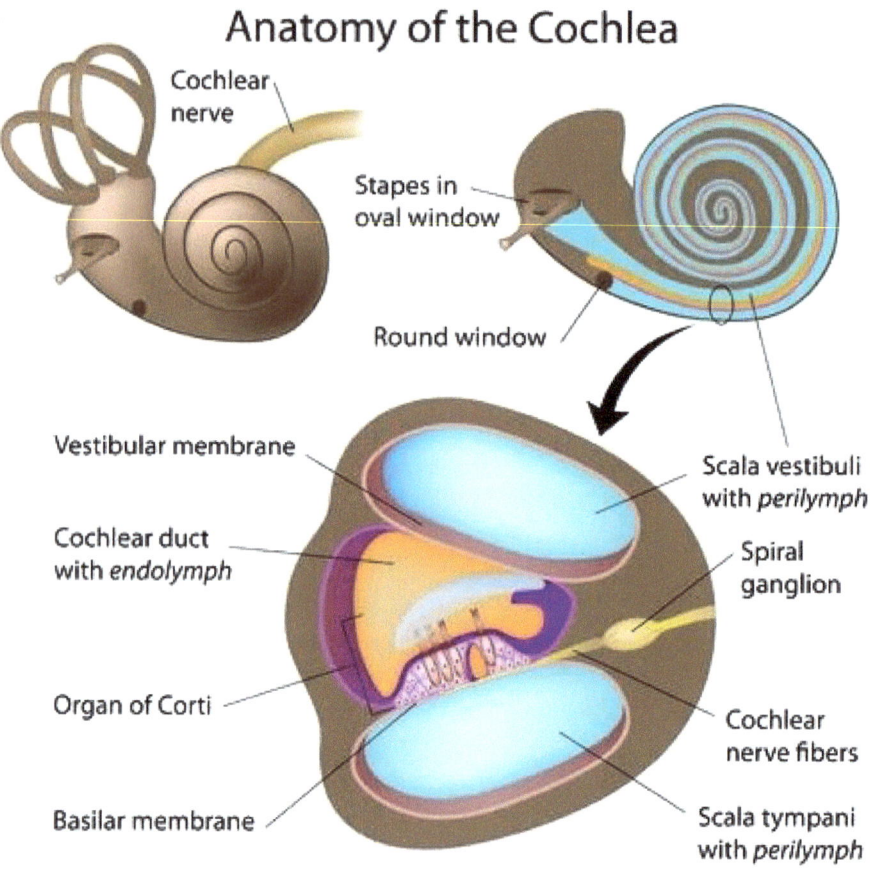

Anatomy of the Cochlea

Cochlear nerve

Stapes in oval window

Round window

Vestibular membrane

Scala vestibuli with *perilymph*

Cochlear duct with *endolymph*

Spiral ganglion

Organ of Corti

Cochlear nerve fibers

Basilar membrane

Scala tympani with *perilymph*

Patients with very severe deafness who cannot benefit even with very powerful hearing aids can be created by cochlear implants. This is where electrodes are implanted in the inner ear.

This is a very expensive procedure and requires intensive speech therapy after the surgery. With technical advances, better cochlear implants are slowly and steadily getting to be available in the market today. These improve hearing considerably. These are also now being recommended for children with severe deafness and mutism.

Mutism

If a child loses his hearing before the age of five, he may also lose the power of speech. And if the child has been born deaf, he will not be able to learn how to speak. Take the example of Helen Keller who became deaf, dumb and blind when a child through scarlet fever.

Luckily, she was fortunate enough to have a good teacher who taught her how to "speak". Speech normally develops by hearing the spoken word. If the deafness is acute, speech is not going to develop.

This is the reason why my student's parents were so terrified that their child was deaf and mute. Testing showed that he was not deaf. In fact, he watched every action being done by his teacher, and laughed on cue, when I was telling theatrical stories to the babies with appropriate gestures, different voices and noises. However, he did not speak, until absolutely necessary and that too to give a peremptory order to his parents!

There are plenty of special schools where such children are educated. Such children can be integrated into normal schools after proper training for a couple of years. Advanced cochlear implants are also being used in such children with very encouraging results.

Preventing Deafness

Deafness, permanent and temporary can be caused due to a large number of reasons, most of which we consider so commonplace that we ignore them. Here are a few precautions which can help prevent ear problems and deafness.

Cleaning of ears

Most of us have got so used to digging our ears with Q-tips or ear buds, because we have seen our parents doing exactly that. Well, if you have the habit of doing that, please do not do so, from now on because you might perforate your eardrum.

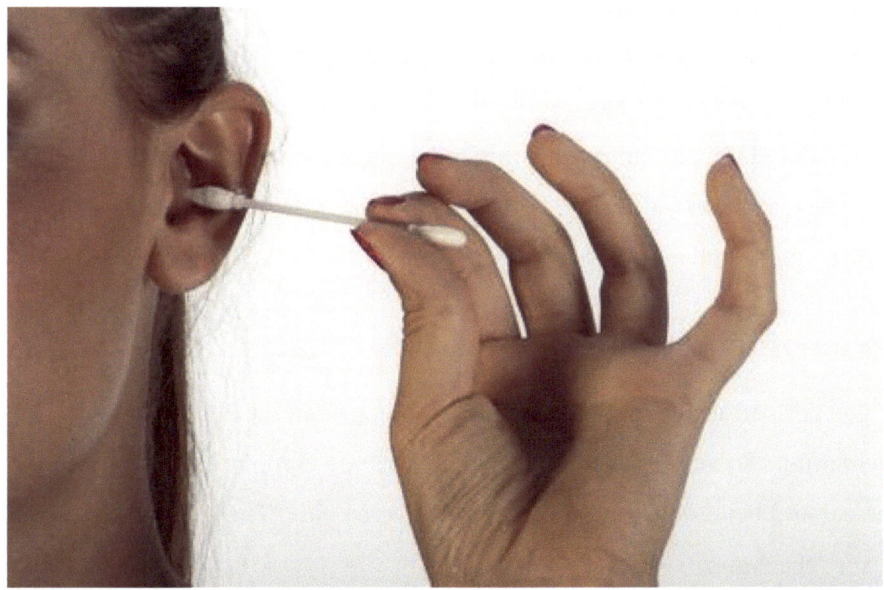

Oh no, you don't!

I also remember once, when my ears were giving me so much trouble at night, that I got an ear bud and put it in my ear. A little bit of gritting of the teeth, and all that infection was out. Unfortunately, when I turned it around to clear the remainder of the infection, the cotton head decided to stay in the inner canal, and to my horror, and dismay, I found myself pulling out just an empty plastic "stick." The cotton bud was fixed right and tight in the ear Canal.

I had enough of good sense not to go poking for it in the ear, with a tweezer, because that would possibly push the cotton right in, and possibly perforate the tympanum.

Naturally, first thing in the morning, I ran to the hospital, where Dr. M got that piece of cotton out, along with accumulated wax and fungus, amid lots of triumphant I told you so's.

So go with my experience, please do not go cleaning out your ears with these earbuds. The ear has a self-cleaning mechanism for wax. All the accumulated wax in the ear is going to be dispelled naturally by itself. However, with self-cleaning, you may push the wax from the outer ears further inside and possibly cause an infection.

Swimming

If you are suffering from any disease or infection in the ear, avoid swimming. To avoid water entering the ear, you can place a cotton bud in the ear and bend down the head on the affected side. The cotton is going to absorb the water.

When I was a child, and I felt that swimming pool water had entered my ears, because there was a "watery" sound in the ear canal, I just lay on my stomach on the bed with my head nearly touching the floor. Then I started moving my jaws, in a masticating action. In a couple of minutes, I could feel the trickle of warm water coming out from the ear canal, down and out, and so this was the way in which I got rid of any accumulated water in the ear canal.

But that did not stop the infections, which would have gone away with a complete bar on swimming for a couple of months.

Loud Sounds

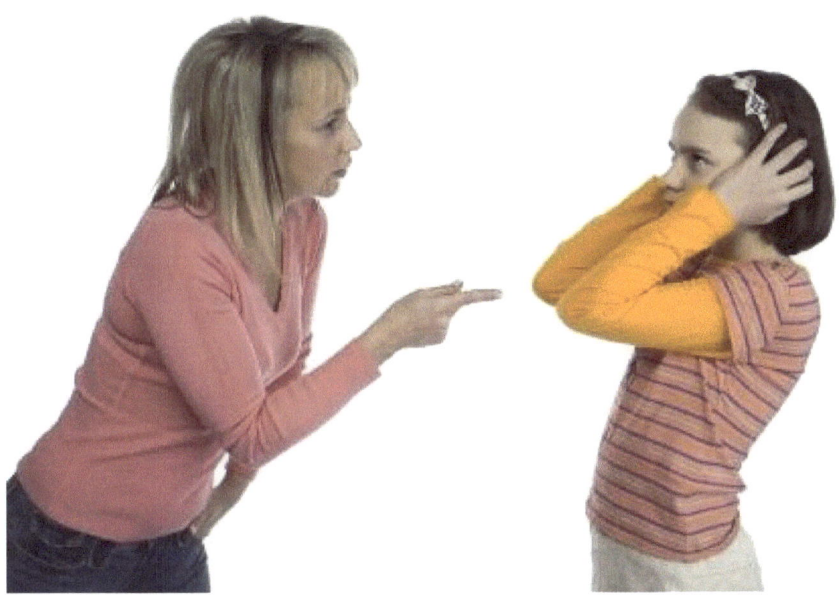

Loud music and loud noises are capable of harming your ears causing temporary or permanent deafness depending on the intensity and the duration of the sound. In the same manner, noise pollution over a long period of time is going to affect your hearing. That is the reason why people working in factories and surrounded by noisy machines are quite capable of saying "huh", when one speaks to them in a softer manner.

High blood pressure and Diabetes

High blood pressure and diabetes are also responsible for damage to the nerves of the ear. These diseases when kept in control can prevent permanent ear damage.

Your Diet

Believe it or not, a fatty diet can affect your hearing, apart from causing fat related diseases in the rest of your body. This is because the walls of blood vessels which are supplying the nerves of ears are thickened with a fatty diet. These are going to cause deafness.

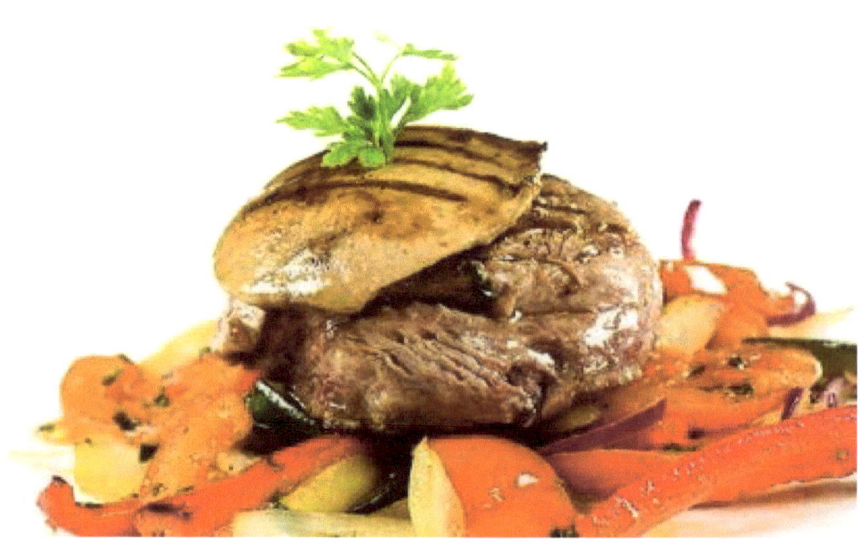

So tempting, but alas, bad for our weight, future health and also ears!

Neglecting a Cold

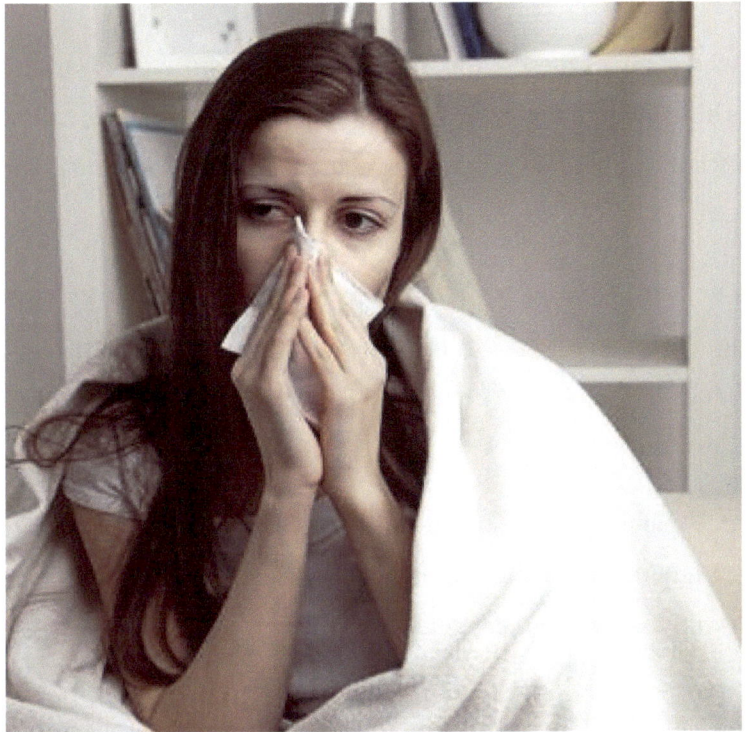

A neglected cold or any sort of infection in the throat could lead to an infection in the middle year through the Eustachian tube which is connected to the ear, along with the nose and throat. In the same manner, if you blow your nose forcibly, this can push a nasal infection into the ear, and infect it.

Genetic Factors

There are number of genetic factors which can also create deafness. These include consanguineous marriages – those which are among close relatives. That is the reason why so inbred Royal families where marriages were between relatives suffered from so many blood related and gene related diseases. That is because they never got a chance to get a healthier bloodstock or bloodline or gene line to strengthen their disease ridden inbred family circle.

That is why many of these aristocrats and royalties suffered from congenital deafness along with other gene related diseases. Also, if the parents suffered from an Rh incompatibility, there was a chance that the offspring would be deaf.

This last scientific discovery of course, was found only in the 20th century, but before that, it was all put down to bad luck and the stars, especially when all the children turned out to be deaf, or suffering from other congenital ailments.

In the same manner, if the expectant mother suffered from German measles, diabetes, high blood pressure, or injury, when she was expecting, her child could possibly suffer from congenital deafness.

Conclusion

This book has given you plenty of information about your ear, and how you can prevent and cure ear problems. There are plenty of natural remedies, with which you can keep your years healthy, especially when you have the feeling that there is plenty of wax accumulated, and how do you get rid of it.

Like I said before, the ear is going to get rid of the wax naturally, but you can speed up the process by softening the wax. This is done by putting a couple of drops of warm almond oil in your ears, before you go to sleep and plug them with cotton.

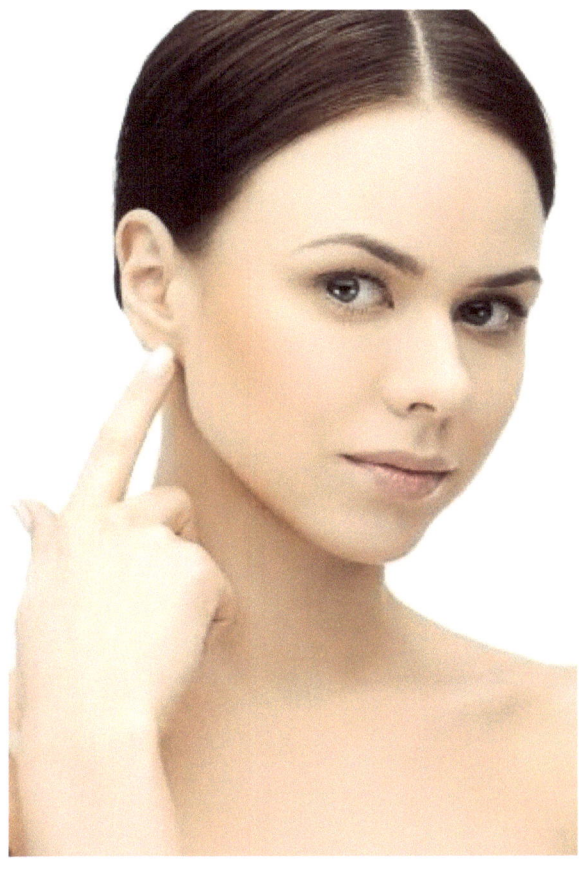

When you wake up the next morning, you are going to find your hearing much clearer. In the same manner, if there was some sort of discharge in the ear , and there was no doctor around, ancient wise women would recommend heating 2 teaspoons full of mustard oil, adding half a teaspoonful of Bishops Weed and two flakes of crushed garlic. These were then boiled until they turned red. These were filtered and then used as ear drops – when cooled to body temperature – until the infection got cured.

In the same manner, if you are suffering from earaches, just makes a few drops of fresh lime juice in one teaspoonful of lukewarm water. Put four drops of this into the affected ear.

These are natural remedies which are time-tested and timeworn, and have been used by people who did not have easy access to hospitals, and antibiotics. So take care of your ears, hear that?

Live Long and Prosper!

Author Bio

Dueep Jyot Singh is a Management and IT Professional who managed to gather Postgraduate qualifications in Management and English and Degrees in Science, French and Education while pursuing different enjoyable career options like being an hospital administrator, IT,SEO and HRD Database Manager/ trainer, movie , radio and TV scriptwriter, theatre artiste and public speaker, lecturer in French, Marketing and Advertising, ex-Editor of Hearts On Fire (now known as Solstice) Books Missouri USA, advice columnist and cartoonist, publisher and Aviation School trainer, ex-moderator on Medico.in, banker, student councilor ,travelogue writer … among other things!

One fine morning, she decided that she had enough of killing herself by Degrees and went back to her first love -- writing. It's more enjoyable! She already has 48 published academic and 14 fiction- in- different- genre books under her belt.

When she is not designing websites or making Graphic design illustrations for clients , she is browsing through old bookshops hunting for treasures, of which she has an enviable collection – including R.L. Stevenson, O.Henry, Dornford Yates, Maurice Walsh, De Maupassant, Victor Hugo, Sapper, C.N. Williamson, "Bartimeus" and the crown of her collection- Dickens "The Old Curiosity Shop," and "Martin Chuzzlewit" and so on… Just call her "Renaissance Woman" - collecting herbal remedies, acting like Universal Helping Hand/Agony Aunt, or escaping to her dear mountains for a bit of exploring, collecting herbs and plants, and trekking.

Check out some of the other JD-Biz Publishing books

Gardening Series on Amazon

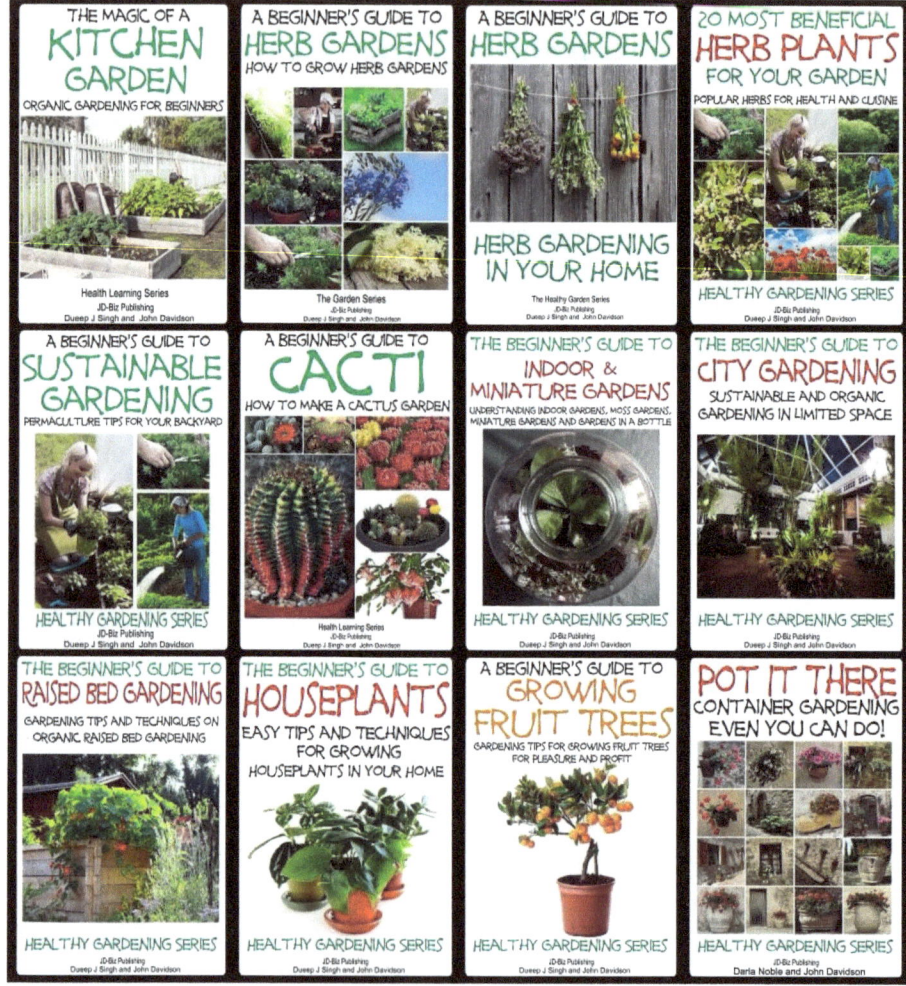

Download Free Books!

http://MendonCottageBooks.com

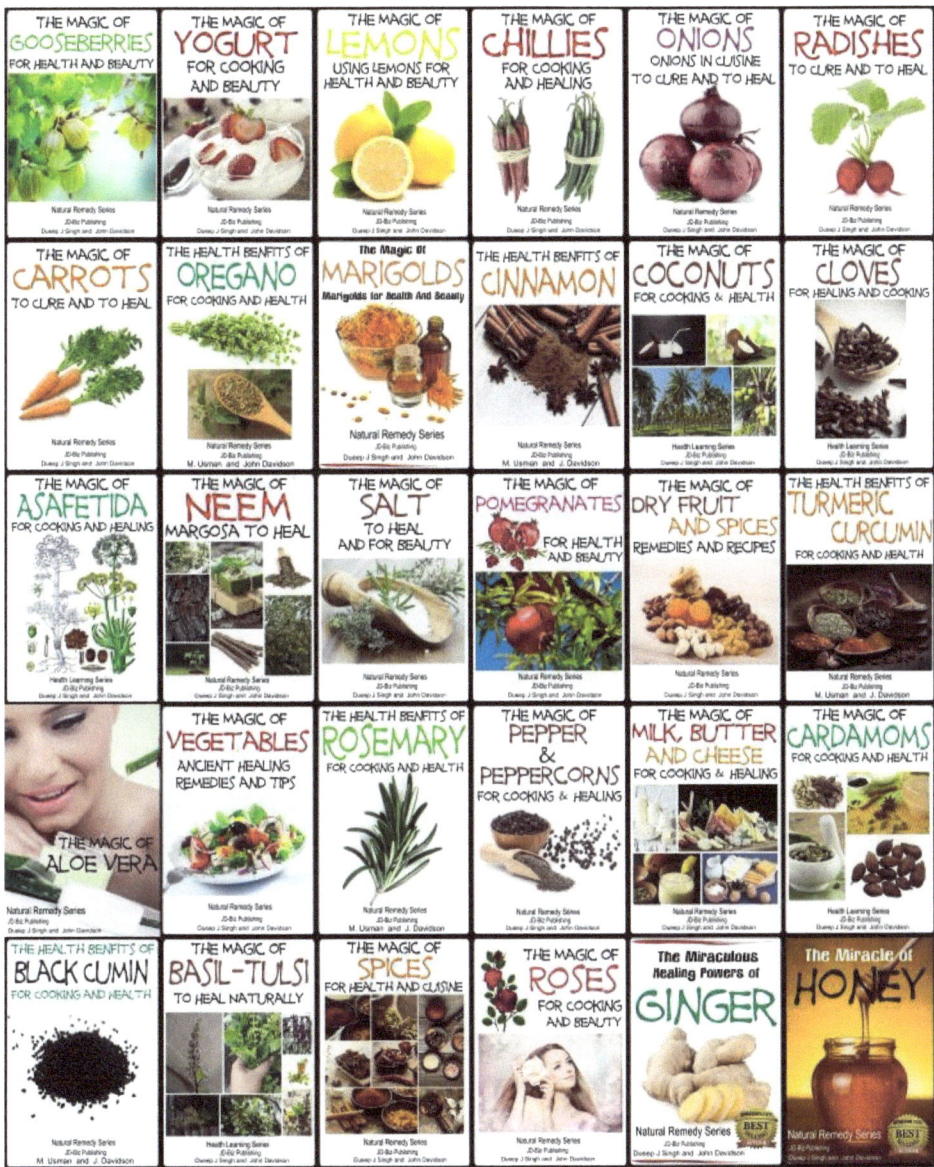

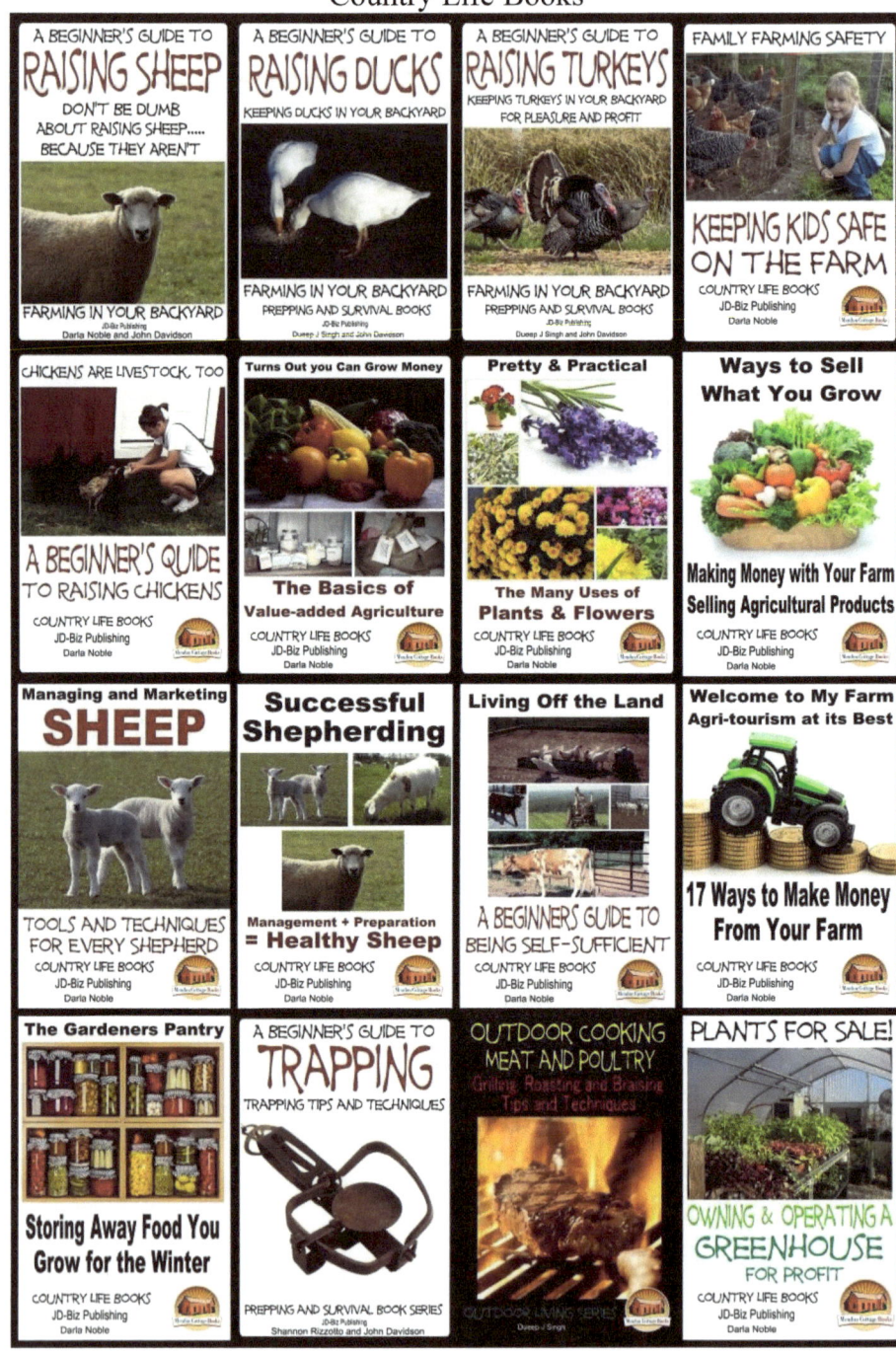

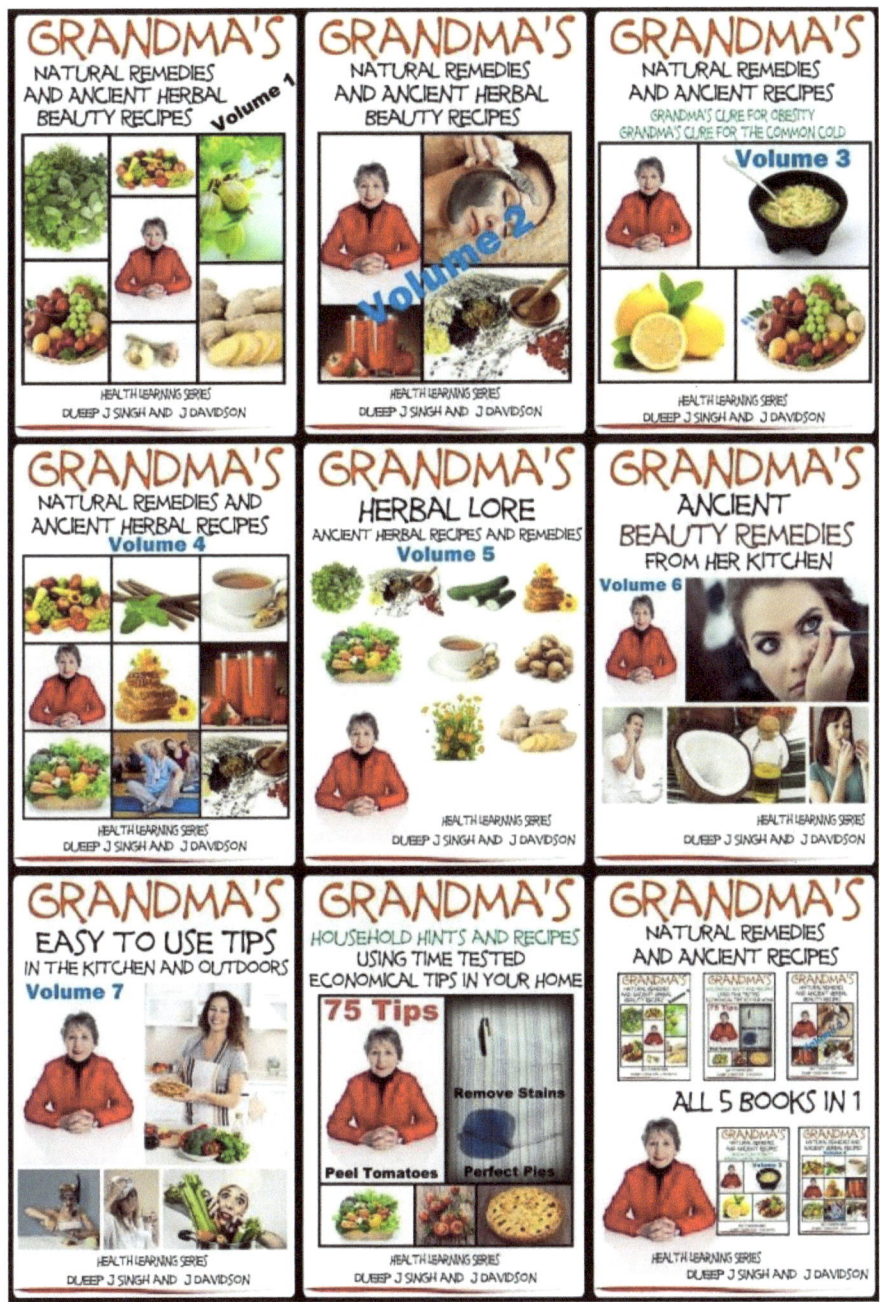

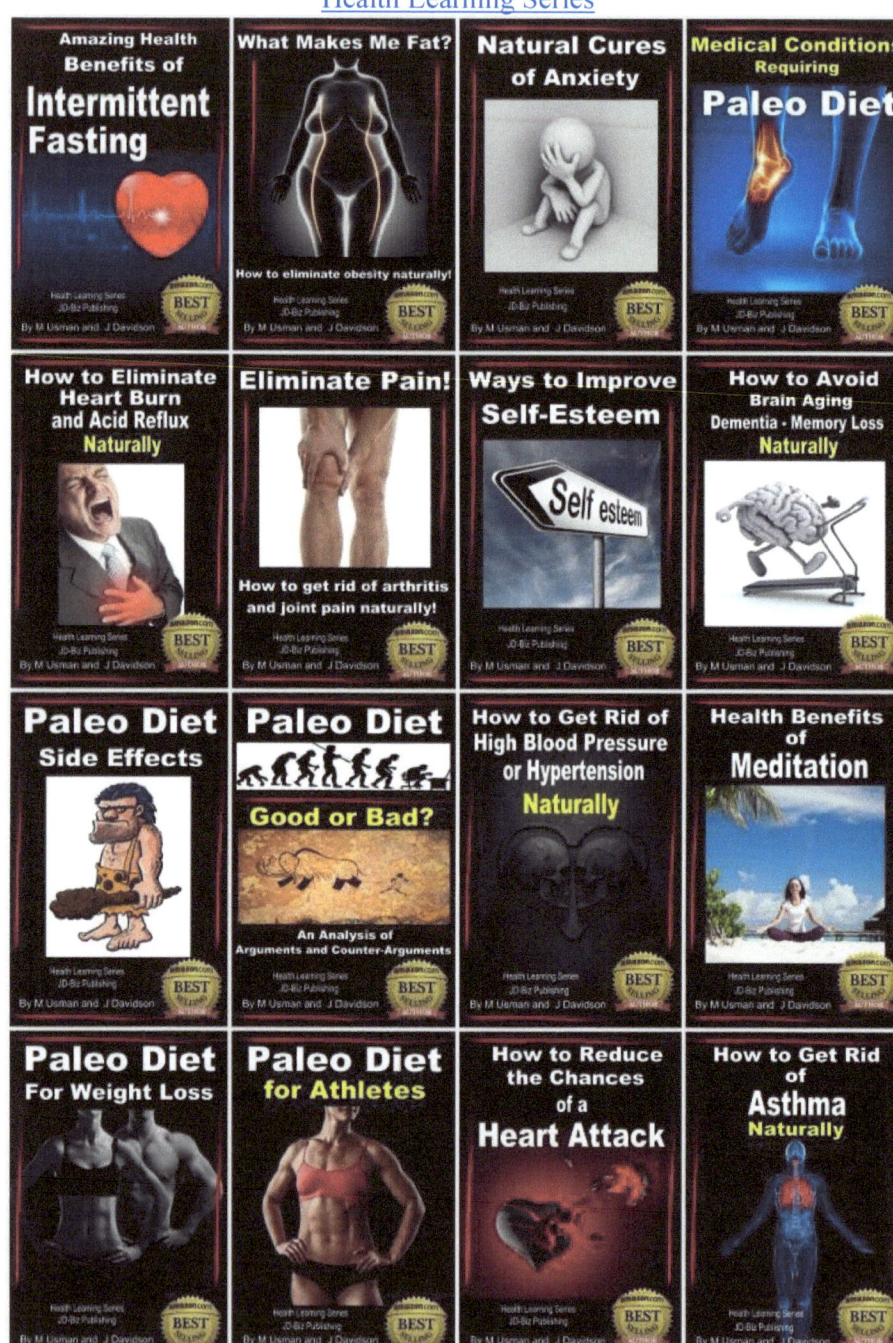

Amazing Animal Book Series

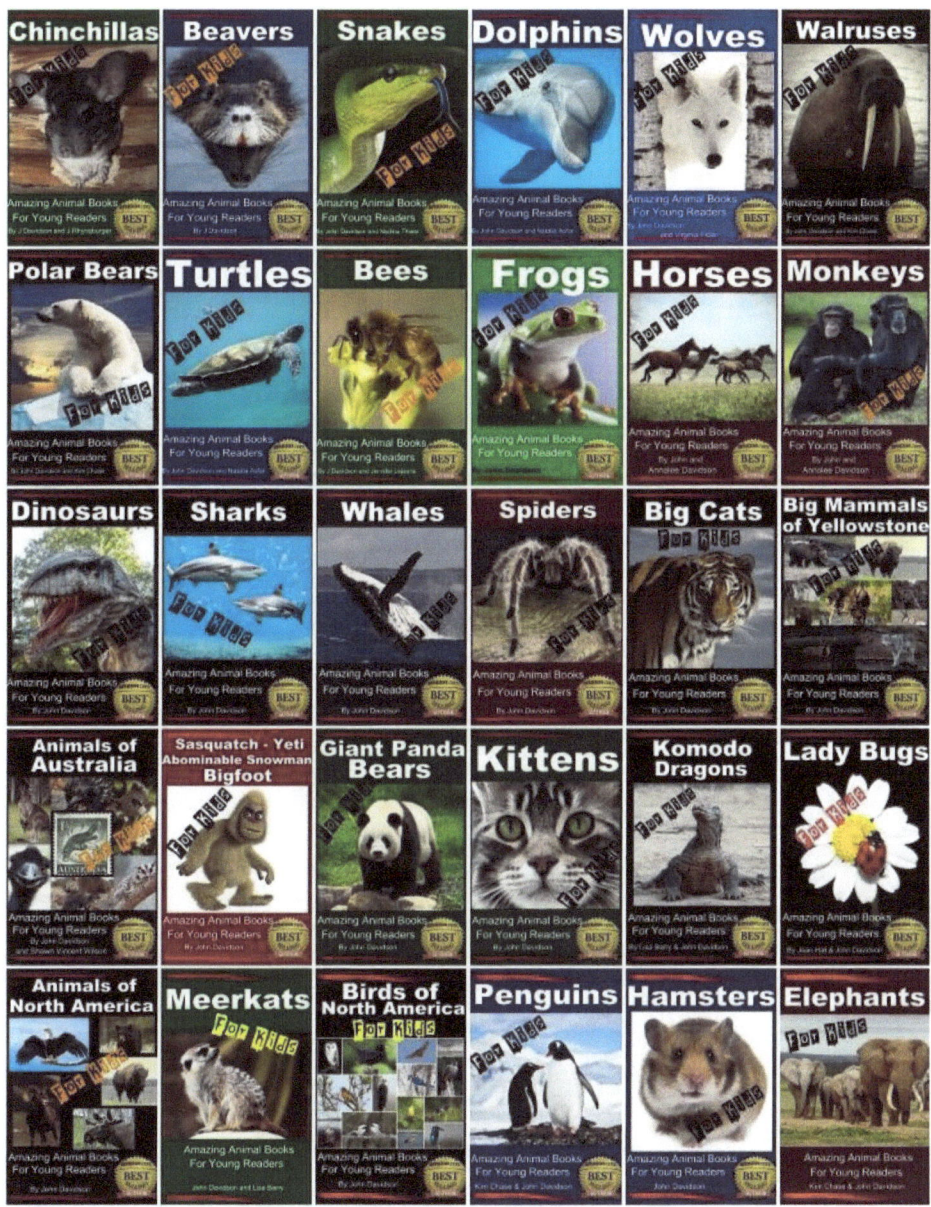

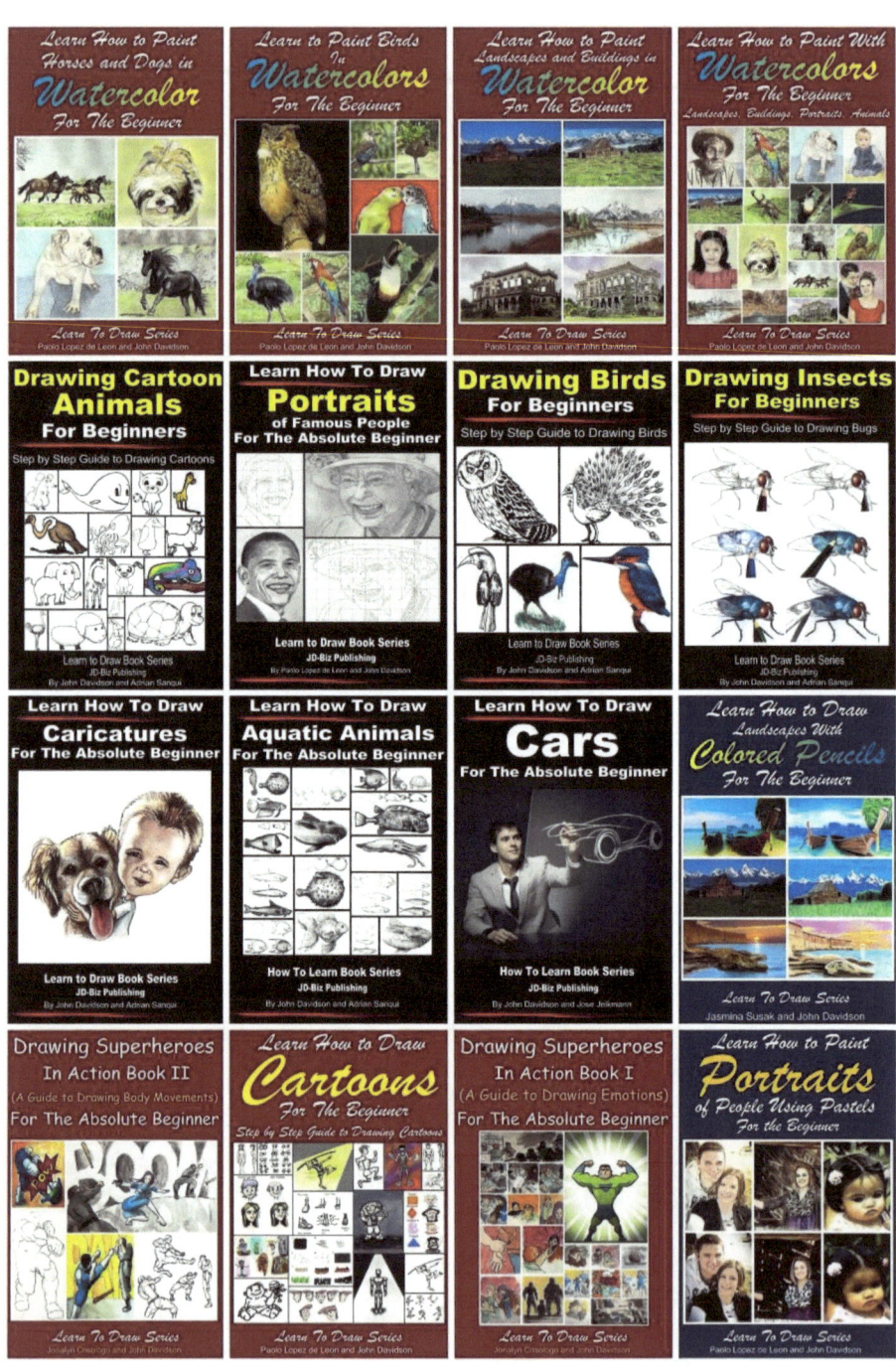

How to Build and Plan Books

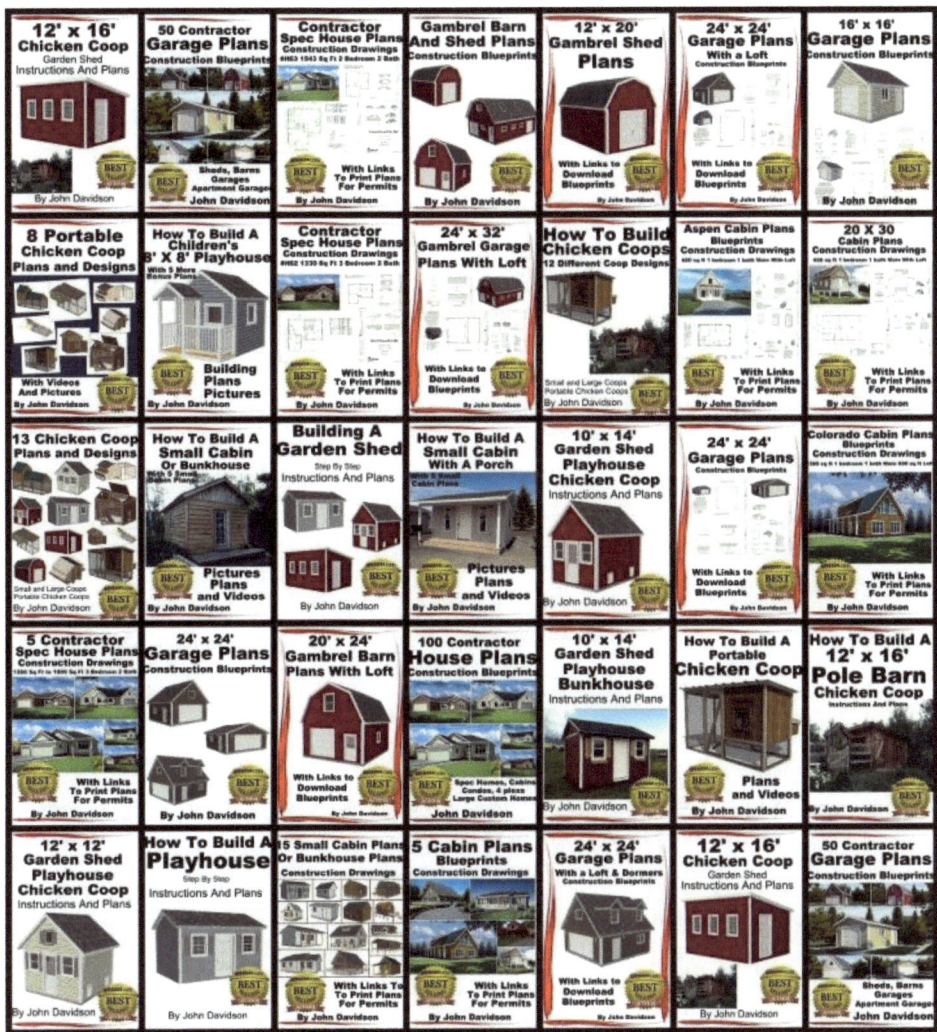

Entrepreneur Book Series

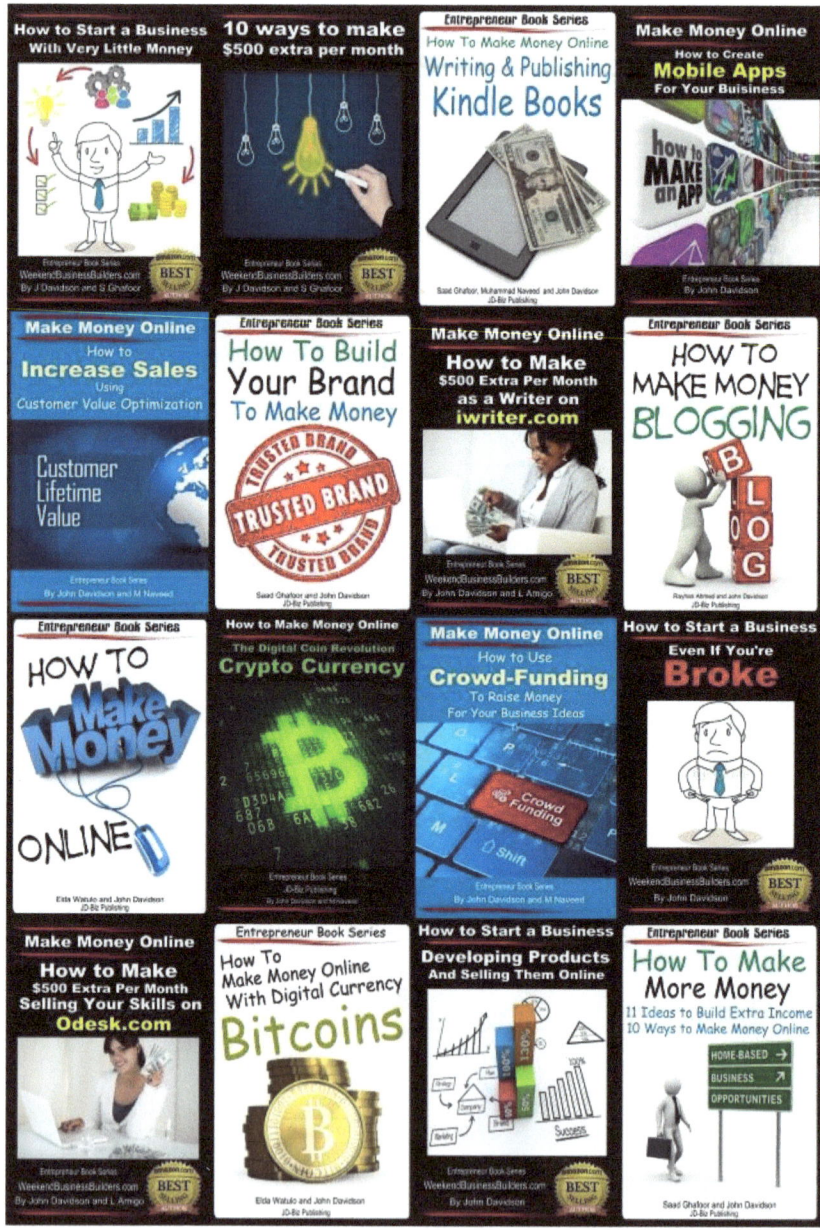

Our books are available at

1. Amazon.com

2. Barnes and Noble

3. Itunes

4. Kobo

5. Smashwords

6. Google Play Books

Download Free Books!

http://MendonCottageBooks.com

Publisher

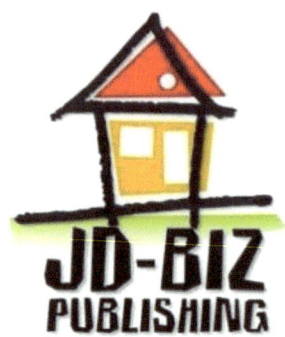

JD-Biz Corp

P O Box 374

Mendon, Utah 84325

http://www.jd-biz.com/

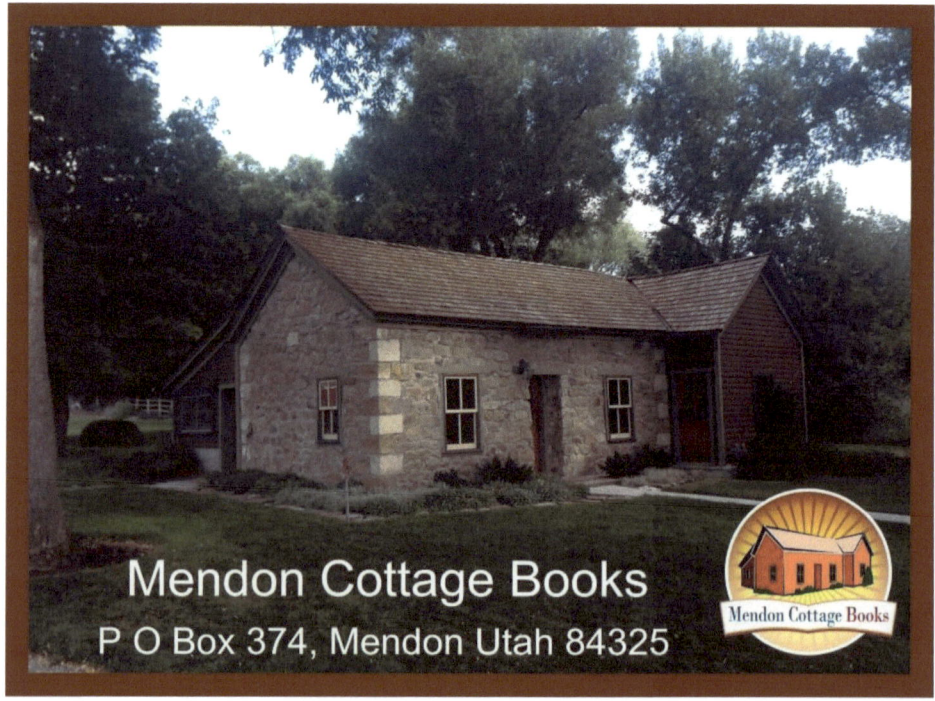

www.ingramcontent.com/pod-product-compliance
Lightning Source LLC
Chambersburg PA
CBHW040315010626
45792CB00022B/335